The Full Body Reset:

"Your Manual for Weight Reduction for a Trim Figure, Ideal Wellbeing, and a Body You'll Cherish Into Midlife"

By

Kevin S. Washington

Table of content

Introduction   5

Chapter 1   7

The anti-aging magic of protein timing   7

The Tale of 2 Healthy Regimens   10

Chapter 2   13

Our changing body, our changing necessities   13

Understanding Muscle Misfortune and Influence Decline:15

The Job of Sustenance in Turning Around Muscle
Misfortune: 16

Chapter Three   19

We should Go through a Day Overall Body Reset   19

7-Day Full Body Reset Test Menu   22

Chapter four: 28

Your Enchanted General Store Name Decoder   28

Full Body Reset Shopping Rundown: 31

Chapter Five   36

Investigating the Entire Body Reset   36

Summary   51

Introduction

Welcome to "The Full Body Reset: Your Manual for Weight Reduction for a Trim Figure, Ideal Wellbeing, and a Body You'll Cherish Into Midlife." In the pages that follow, leave on a groundbreaking excursion that rises above regular weight reduction counsel. This isn't simply one more eating routine book; it's an extensive aide intended to engage you with the information and devices required for supportable change.

In a world immersed with clashing well-being data, "The Full Body Reset" stands apart as your dependable friend, grounded in proof-based methodologies and master bits of knowledge. We're not promising convenient solutions or one-size-fits-all arrangements; all things considered, we're welcoming you to embrace a comprehensive methodology that tends to the actual parts of weight the executives as well as the essential association among psyche and body.

All through these parts, you'll investigate customized nourishment plans, powerful workout schedules, and the meaning of mental prosperity in your weight reduction venture. This guide goes past the shallow journey for a trim figure; about developing a way of life that upholds your general well-being and life span.

Whether you're simply beginning your wellness way or looking for a midlife reset, "The Full Body Reset" offers reasonable guidance, significant stages, and a guide to a better, more dynamic you. Now is the right time to break liberated from the pattern of brief arrangements and leave on an excursion that prompts enduring change.

Prepare to rediscover your body's true capacity, embrace ideal well-being, and become hopelessly enamored with the mind-boggling vessel that brings you through midlife and then some. This isn't simply a book; it's your solicitation to a more full, better life.

Chapter 1

The anti-aging magic of protein timing

Protein timing is an acknowledged practice among numerous competitors, jocks, and standard individuals hoping to acquire muscle, however, the science is nowhere near definitive. Timing protein implies eating it at specific seasons of day to augment benefits e.g expanded bulk

Lacking protein consumption for the more seasoned grown-ups adds to a diminishing for possible later use limit, expanded skin delicacy, diminished safe capability, less fortunate mending, and longer recovery from disease.

Timing protein consumption decisively, particularly around feasts and active work, can augment its viability. Consuming protein-rich dinners uniformly over the day invigorates muscle protein combination, the procedure vital for muscle support and fixing.

This is particularly significant for the old, as it checks the regular decrease in muscle protein union related to maturing protein, the structure block of life, becomes the overwhelming focus in the counter maturing account, displaying its significant job in muscle maintenance, digestion, and general cell wellbeing. Understanding the cooperative energy between the right protein sources and vital timing discloses an amazing asset in challenging the maturing system.

1. Muscle Maintenance: As we age, protecting bulk turns out to be progressively urgent for keeping up with strength and portability. The right protein sources, wealthy in fundamental amino acids, are instrumental in advancing muscle protein blend. Excellent proteins, like lean meats, fish, eggs, and plant-based choices like quinoa or tofu, give the amino corrosive profile important to help and remake muscle tissue. Consuming these protein sources in a calculated manner, particularly post-practice or over the day, turns into a foundation for protecting and fabricating slender bulk, critical in the fight against age-related muscle misfortune.

2. Digestion boost: Protein has a thermogenic impact on the body, meaning it requires more energy to be utilized contrasted with fats or carbs. This expanded metabolic rate supports weight the board as well as turns out to be more critical with age when digestion will in general stop. Integrating protein into dinners and bites can add to keeping a sound weight and supporting metabolic capability.

This is especially significant as it mitigates the normal decrease in metabolic rate that frequently goes with the maturing system.

3. Cell Wellbeing:

Proteins are the designers of cell structures, affecting everything from safe capability to DNA fixes. The right protein sources supply the body with fundamental amino acids, supporting the union of compounds, chemicals, and antibodies basic for ideal cell wellbeing. Moreover, certain proteins contain bioactive peptides, adding to cancer prevention agents and calming impacts that battle cell stress and harm. By picking supplement-thick protein sources like fish, nuts, and vegetables, people can emphatically affect cell well-being, possibly dialing back the maturing system at the sub-atomic level.

4. Tactical Timing:

Timing matters about protein utilization. Disseminating protein consumption equitably over the day guarantees a consistent inventory of amino acids, advancing muscle protein union and keeping a positive nitrogen balance. Consolidating protein-rich feasts or bites, particularly post-workout, improves recuperation and muscle transformation. This essential methodology upholds muscle maintenance as well as advances the metabolic reaction, adding to by and large imperativeness.

The Tale of 2 Healthy Regimens

Quite a long time ago in the curious town of Wellsville, two companions, Emma and Oliver, set out on an excursion to find the mysteries of a solid and energetic life through the force of their eating regimens.

Emma, a nutrition enthusiast, embraced a plant-put-together eating regimen that flourished concerning brilliant vegetables, entire grains, and vegetables.

Her mornings started with a dynamic smoothie bowl, overflowing with berries, kale, and a sprinkle of chia seeds.

For lunch, she partook in a good quinoa salad stacked with broiled vegetables and finished off with a fiery vinaigrette.

Emma's meals were a festival of flavors, highlighting dishes like lentil curry or yam tacos.

Oliver, then again, was a firm backer of the Mediterranean eating regimen.

His days began with a comfortable breakfast of entire-grain toast, avocado, and a shower of olive oil.

For lunch, he relished an exemplary Greek plate of mixed greens with feta, olives, and a variety of new tomatoes and cucumbers.

Suppers were a magnificent undertaking with barbecued fish, prepared with spices, and joined by a side of quinoa and sautéed greens.

As the seasons changed in Wellsville, Emma, and Oliver encountered the significant effect of their picked diets. Emma ended up overflowing with energy, because of the supplement-rich plant-based food sources that energized her day. Her skin shined, and she felt a feeling of essentialness that rose above simple actual well-being.

In the meantime, Oliver savored the heart-solid advantages of his Mediterranean eating routine. The omega-3 unsaturated fats from fish and the cell reinforcements from olive oil added to his general prosperity. His cholesterol levels were under tight restraints, and he wondered about the flexibility of his heart.

One radiant evening, Emma and Oliver chose to have a local area feast, exhibiting the tasty potential outcomes of their separate eating regimens. The town square changed into a bright exhibit of dishes, with Emma's plant-based manifestations blending with Oliver's Mediterranean joys.

As the residents accumulated, they delighted in the happy environment, relishing the different and nutritious contributions.

 The occasion turned into an impetus for a better local area, motivating others to investigate the advantages of various weight control plans and find what turned out best for them.

In Wellsville, the story of Emma and Oliver turned into a legend — an update that there is not a one-size-fits-all way to deal with a solid eating routine. All things being equal, the critical lies in embracing assorted, supplement-thick food varieties that line up with individual inclinations and advance general prosperity. Thus, the inhabitants of Wellsville proceeded with their excursion towards wellbeing, directed by the insight of Emma's plant-based enjoyments and Oliver's Mediterranean fortunes.

The ideal protein sources at the perfect minute arise as a powerful power chasing opposing the maturing system. From protecting bulk to helping digestion and sustaining cell wellbeing, protein turns into a vital partner in advancing a strong and dynamic body all through the excursion of life.

Chapter 2

Our changing body, our changing necessities

As we smoothly cross the excursion of life, our bodies go through a progression of changes. From the richness of youth to the insight of midlife, understanding the nuanced shifts in our physiology becomes foremost in making a maintainable way towards ideal well-being and a trim figure.

1. Embracing the Progression of Time: Our bodies are wonders of transformation, and as time passes, they go through changes that require a recalibration of our way of dealing with well-being. In this part, we dive into the complexities of maturing — embracing the insight that accompanies it and recognizing the remarkable requirements our bodies foster over the long haul. As the scene of our physiology develops, so should our techniques for weighing the executives and in general prosperity.

2. Hormonal Agreement: One of the focal subjects in the midlife venture is the rhythmic movement of chemicals.

Understanding what hormonal changes mean for digestion, bulk, and generally speaking body arrangement is vital to exploring this stage with artfulness. From variances in estrogen to changes in testosterone levels, we investigate how hormonal congruity assumes a critical part in the Full Body Reset.

3. Adjusting Sustenance to Midlife Needs: Midlife carries with it an unmistakable arrangement of wholesome prerequisites. We unwind the secret of how our dietary requirements develop, stressing the significance of supplement-thick food varieties that take care of our changing digestion and back muscle maintenance. From bone well-being to heart well-being, find the supplements that become fundamental on this groundbreaking excursion.

4. Practice Reconsidered: Practice is a deep-rooted friend, yet its structure and center shift as we age. This page acquaints a rethought approach to wellness, integrating exercises that shape our constitution as well as improve joint adaptability, bone thickness, and cardiovascular well-being. Whether it's embracing yoga for its brain-body association or integrating strength to prepare for bone thickness, we investigate practices that take care of our evolving needs.

5. The Psyche Body Association: Midlife isn't simply an actual change; it's a comprehensive recalibration.

 In this section, we dive into the significant association between psychological wellness and actual prosperity. Stress the executives, care, and the force of a positive outlook become the overwhelming focus as we perceive the cooperative connection between our psychological and actual selves.

Understanding Muscle Misfortune and Influence Decline:

the continuous loss of bulk, otherwise called sarcopenia. This decline normally starts around the age of 30, with a more articulated impact as we enter our 40s and 50s. Sarcopenia is joined by a decrease in muscle strength and power, affecting our capacity to perform everyday exercises and keep up with in general actual capability.

The maturing system adds to this muscle misfortune through different instruments. Hormonal changes, particularly a decrease in the development of chemical and testosterone levels, assume a part in reducing muscle union. Moreover, there's an expansion in irritation, oxidative pressure, and a decrease in cell fix systems, all of which add to the breakdown of muscle tissue after some time.

The Job of Sustenance in Turning Around Muscle Misfortune:

Legitimate substance arises as an incredible asset to neutralize the impacts of muscle misfortune and declining influence related to maturing. Here is a nitty gritty investigation of how sustenance can switch this cycle:

1. Protein's Urgent Job: Protein turns into a foundation in the fight against sarcopenia. Satisfactory protein admission, especially wealthy in fundamental amino acids, upholds muscle protein amalgamation. Lean sources like poultry, fish, eggs, and plant-based choices like vegetables and tofu give the fundamental structure blocks to keeping up with and fixing muscle tissue. Dispersing protein consumption equally over the day guarantees a consistent stockpile of amino acids, advancing muscle well-being.

2. Leucine and Muscle Union: Leucine, a fundamental amino corrosive bountiful in specific food varieties like meat, dairy, and soy, assumes an urgent part in invigorating muscle protein combinations. Remembering leucine-rich food varieties for the eating regimen becomes critical for maturing people hoping to safeguard and modify bulk. Spread chain amino corrosive enhancements can likewise be considered to upgrade leucine admission, underlining their expected job in fighting muscle misfortune.

3. Opposition Preparing and Protein Cooperative energy: While legitimate nourishment is fundamental, its belongings are potentiated when joined with obstruction preparation. Taking part in customary strength-preparing practices makes a synergistic relationship with protein consumption, boosting muscle muscle-protein combination. This blend is especially viable in turning around age-related muscle misfortune, improving strength, and reestablishing influence.

4. Micronutrients for Muscle Wellbeing: Past macronutrients, and satisfactory admission of micronutrients like vitamin D, calcium, and omega-3 unsaturated fats become significant for keeping up with muscle and bone well-being. These supplements add to general outer muscle respectability, decreasing the gamble of breaks and upgrading actual capability.

5. Hydration and Muscle Capability: Legitimate hydration is frequently disregarded yet assumes a fundamental part in muscle capability. Lack of hydration can debilitate actual execution and worsen muscle exhaustion. Guaranteeing a sufficient water admission upholds muscle capability and keeps up with by and large actual execution, particularly in more seasoned people.

All in all, the maturing system might achieve muscle misfortune and a decrease in influence, however with a key and healthfully sound methodology, these impacts can be relieved. Through an eating routine rich in protein, leucine, and fundamental supplements, joined with designated obstruction preparation, people can switch the tide of muscle misfortune, recover influence, and partake more dynamically and satisfyingly of life as they age. The excursion towards ideal muscle well-being starts with our decisions on our plates and reaches out to the energetic and strong lives we lead.

Chapter Three

We should Go through a Day Overall Body Reset

Set out on a day-long excursion that exemplifies the embodiment of the Full Body Reset — a complete manual for recalibrating your way of life for supported weight reduction, ideal well-being, and a body you'll cherish well into midlife.

Morning Schedule: Stimulating the Body and Brain

1. Awaken with Hydration: Begin your day by rehydrating your body. A glass of water with a sprinkle of lemon launches hydration as well as gives an invigorating explosion of L-ascorbic acid.

2. Careful Development or Extending: Take part in delicate stretches or a short care schedule. This establishes an inspirational vibe for the afternoon, improving adaptability, and advancing mental lucidity.

3. Protein-Pressed Breakfast: Kick off your digestion with a protein-rich breakfast. Whether it's a generous omelet with vegetables or a plant-based protein smoothie, guarantee your most memorable feast is a supplement thick force to be reckoned with.

Early Afternoon Sustenance: Powering Your Body for Progress

4. Nibble Shrewd: Battle early in the day craving with a modest bite. Pick a small bunch of nuts, a piece of natural product, or Greek yogurt to keep energy levels stable.

5. Lunch for Supported Energy: Make a lunch that adjusts lean proteins, entire grains, and beautiful vegetables. A quinoa salad with barbecued chicken or a chickpea bowl with dynamic veggies gives supported energy without the mid-evening droop.

Evening Renewal: Reinforcing the Body and Psyche

6. Remain Hydrated: Keep on focusing on hydration over the day. Home-grown teas, implanted water, or even some green tea offer cell reinforcements and add to by and large prosperity.

7. Move with Reason: Integrate development into your evening. Whether it's an energetic walk, a short exercise meeting, or a progression of the work area, keep your body dynamic to help disseminate mental concentration.

8. Careful Breaks: Enjoy short reprieves to rehearse care or profound relaxation. These snapshots of respite add to pressure decrease and advance a positive outlook.

Evening Reclamation: Supporting and Planning for Rest

9. Adjusted Supper:: Finish up your day with an even supper. Consolidate lean proteins, entire grains, and different vegetables to give fundamental supplements to recuperation and muscle wellbeing.

10. Careful Eating: Practice careful eating during supper. Relish each nibble, focusing on appetite and totality prompts. This cultivates a sound connection with food and energizes better processing.

11. Hydrate with Natural Tea: Wind down the night with a quieting natural tea. This guides in hydration as well as supports unwinding, setting up your body for a helpful night's rest.

Evening time Ceremonies: Guaranteeing Quality Rest

12. Screen Detox: Limit screen time before bed to advance the development of melatonin, and the rest chemicals. Participate in quieting exercises like perusing a book or rehearsing delicate extending.

13. Rest Inciting Tidbit (Discretionary): If hungry before bed, pick a little, rest prompting nibble like a modest bunch of almonds or a piece of turkey. These tidbits contain tryptophan, advancing unwinding and supporting a more peaceful rest.

7-Day Full Body Reset Test Menu

Day 1:

Breakfast:

* Fried eggs with spinach and tomatoes, entire grain toast, and a side of berries.

Lunch:

* Barbecued chicken plate of mixed greens with blended greens, quinoa, cherry tomatoes, cucumbers, and a lemon vinaigrette.

Snacks:

* Greek yogurt with a sprinkle of chia seeds and a little small bunch of almonds.

Supper:

* Prepared salmon with simmered yams and steamed broccoli.

Day 2:

Breakfast:

* Smoothie with kale, banana, Greek yogurt, and a scoop of protein powder.

Lunch:

* Lentil soup with a side of entire grain wafers and a blended green serving of mixed greens.

Snacks:

* Apple cuts with almond spread.

Supper:

* Sautéed tofu with blended vegetables and quinoa.

Day 3:

Breakfast:

* Oats finished off with cut strawberries, pecans, and a shower of honey.

Lunch:

* Turkey and avocado wrap with an entire grain tortilla, presented with a side of carrot sticks.

Snacks:

* Curds with pineapple pieces.

Supper:

* Barbecued shrimp with earthy-colored rice and sautéed asparagus.

Day 4:

Breakfast:

* Entire grain flapjacks finished off with Greek yogurt and blended berries.

Lunch:

* Quinoa salad with dark beans, corn, cherry tomatoes, and a lime-cilantro dressing.

Snacks:

* Modest bunch of blended nuts and dried natural products.

Supper:

* Chicken bosom with yam wedges and a side of cooked Brussels sprouts.

Day 5:

Breakfast:

* Vegetable omelet with entire grain toast and cut oranges.

Lunch:

* Chickpea and vegetable pan-fried food with earthy-colored rice.

Snacks:

* Curds and cut peaches.

Supper:

* Prepared cod with quinoa pilaf and steamed green beans.

Day 6:

Breakfast:

* Chia seed pudding with almond milk, finished off with new berries.

Lunch:

* Spinach and feta-stuffed chicken bosom with a side of broiled yams.

Snacks:

* Greek yogurt parfait with granola and blended natural products.

Supper:

* Turkey stew with dark beans, served over a bed of earthy-colored rice.

Day 7:

Breakfast:

* Entire grain toast with crushed avocado, poached eggs, and a side of grapefruit.

Lunch:

* Quinoa bowl with barbecued vegetables, chickpeas, and a tahini dressing.

Snacks:

* Cut apple with a bit of peanut butter.

Supper:

* Heated chicken thighs with quinoa and a brilliant blended vegetable variety.

Chapter four:

Your Enchanted General Store Name Decoder

In the maze of general store passageways, unraveling food marks turns into craftsmanship, expertise that enables you to pursue informed decisions on your excursion to a Full Body Reset. This part discloses the insider facts behind the names, directing you on the most proficient method to explore the supermarket with certainty, guaranteeing the things you pick to add to weight reduction, ideal well-being, and a body you'll cherish well into midlife.

1. Figuring out the Supplement Code:

Unwind the secrets of sustenance marks by figuring out the key parts. Figure out how to recognize the serving size, calories, and macronutrients per serving. This disentangling system enables you to settle on cognizant choices lined up with your well-being and weight reduction objectives.

2. Be careful with Stowed away Sugars: Sugar frequently hides under different names on fixing records. Expose these assumed names and recognize between normal sugars and added sugars. Your mark decoder prepares you to go with decisions that limit sugar admission, advancing stable energy levels and decreasing the gamble of irritation.

3. Dominating Part Control: Segment sizes assume a critical part in overseeing caloric admission. Figure out how to decipher segment data on names and use it as a manual for forestall overconsumption. Your name decoder turns into an important device in maintaining harmony between extravagance and control.

4. Recognizing Sound Fats: Not all fats are made equivalent. Explore through the sorts of fats recorded on marks, recognizing soaked, unsaturated, and trans fats. Your name decoder helps you in picking items that add to heart well-being and general prosperity.

5. Fresh Experiences into Sugars: Sugars come in different structures, and your mark decoder reveals the qualifications. Separate among mind-boggling and straightforward carbs, stressing entire grains and fiber-rich choices. This ability helps with keeping up with consistent glucose levels and supporting stomach-related well-being.

6. Revealing Protein Ability: Comprehend the protein content of food items and perceive the wellspring of protein. Your mark decoder guides you in picking things rich in excellent proteins, fundamental for muscle maintenance, digestion, and by and large body creation.

7. Interpreting Fixing Records: Fixing records gives a guide to what you're genuinely consuming. Handle the craft of perusing these rundowns, recognizing likely allergens, added substances, and additives. Your name decoder changes you into an insightful customer, settling on items with healthy, conspicuous fixings.

8. Spotting Supplement Rich Food sources: Embrace the capacity to recognize supplement thick food varieties rapidly. Your name decoder guides you towards things loaded with nutrients, minerals, and cancer prevention agents — fundamental components for ideal well-being and imperativeness.

9. Assessing Wellbeing Cases: Explore through the labyrinth of wellbeing claims on bundling. Figure out how to recognize showcasing methodologies and validated medical advantages. Your mark decoder guarantees that items line up with your Full Body Reset objectives as opposed to surrendering to deluding claims.

10. Making a Shopping Rundown for Progress:

Furnished with your name decoder, make a shopping list that focuses on supplement thick, entire food varieties. Change your basic food item stumbles into key undertakings, cultivating a climate at home that upholds your excursion towards a trim figure and ideal well-being.

Full Body Reset Shopping Rundown:

Proteins:

1. Skinless poultry (chicken, turkey)

2. Lean cuts of meat and pork

3. Fish (salmon, fish, mackerel)

4. Tofu or tempeh

5. Eggs

6. Vegetables (lentils, chickpeas, dark beans)

Dairy and Choices:

7. Greek yogurt (unsweetened)

8. Low-fat or plant-based milk (almond, coconut, oat)

9. Curds

Entire Grains:

10. Quinoa

11. Earthy colored rice

12. Entire wheat pasta

13. Oats (rolled or steel-cut)

14. Grain

Vegetables:

15. Salad greens (spinach, kale, arugula)

16. Cruciferous vegetables (broccoli, cauliflower, Brussels sprouts)

17. Brilliant vegetables (ringer peppers, carrots, tomatoes)

18. Avocado

Organic products:

19. Berries (blueberries, strawberries, raspberries)

20. Apples

21. Oranges or grapefruits

22. Bananas

Nuts and Seeds:

23. Almonds

24. Pecans

25. Chia seeds

26. Flaxseeds

Solid Fats:

27. Olive oil

28. Avocado oil

29. Coconut oil

Spices and Flavors:

30. Turmeric

31. Ginger

32. Garlic

33. Cinnamon

34. Basil, cilantro, or parsley

Sans dairy Proteins:

35. Plant-based protein powder

36. Almond or peanut butter (unsweetened)

Fish (if material):

37. Shrimp

38. Cod

39. Mussels

Entire Food Varieties Tidbits:

40. Hummus

41. Veggie sticks (carrots, celery)

42. Blended nuts and seeds

Hydration:

43. Water

44. Home-grown teas

45. Green tea

Fixings and Flavor Enhancers (with some restraint):

46. Mustard

47. Hot sauce

48. Balsamic vinegar

49. Low-sodium soy sauce

Sugars (with some restraint):

50. Honey or maple syrup

By excelling at perusing sustenance realities, you engage yourself to settle on decisions that line up with the standards of the Full Body Reset. This expertise not only backs your prompt well-being and weight reduction objectives but also adds to a manageable and energetic way of life well into midlife. Keep in mind, that each name is a device directing you toward a better, more educated relationship with food.

Chapter Five

Investigating the Entire Body Reset

Setting out on the Full Body Reset venture is a groundbreaking undertaking, yet like any tremendous change, difficulties might emerge. In this part, we address normal detours and give functional answers for investigating your Full Body Reset, guaranteeing you keep on track toward a trim figure, ideal well-being, and a body you'll cherish well into midlife.

1. Leveling Weight reduction:

Issue:

Stagnation in weight reduction progress.

Arrangement:

Rethink your calorie admission, change segment measures, or alter your workout daily schedule. Bring assortment into exercises and consider talking with a nutritionist to refine your dietary arrangement.

2. Close to home Eating:

Issue:

Going to nourishment for solace or stress alleviation.

Arrangement:

Foster elective survival techniques like care, contemplation, or taking part in leisure activities. Distinguish close-to-home triggers and address them straightforwardly instead of depending on nourishment for profound satisfaction.

3. Absence of Inspiration:

Issue:

Battling to remain spurred in your Full Body Reset venture.

Arrangement:

Return to your underlying objectives, celebrate little triumphs, and help yourself to remember the advantages accomplished up to this point. Think about tracking down an exercise mate or looking for help from loved ones.

4. Stomach-related Distress:

Issue:

Experience bulging, gas, or acid reflux.

Arrangement:

Assess your fiber admission and progressively increment it to permit your stomach-related framework to adjust. Remain hydrated, bite food completely, and consider consolidating your stomach well disposed food varieties like yogurt and aged choices.

5. Conflicting Rest Examples:

Issue:

Unpredictable rest influences generally speaking prosperity.

Arrangement:

Lay out a reliable rest schedule, limit screen time before bed, and establish a loosening-up sleep time climate. Focus on quality rest as it assumes a vital part in weight the board and generally wellbeing.

6. Prevalent difficulties and Occasions:

Issue:

Exploring social circumstances and occasions that spin around unfortunate food decisions.

Arrangement:

Prepare, impart your dietary inclinations, and carry a dish that lines up with your Full Body Reset. Center around mingling as opposed to exclusively on food, and practice balance whenever confronted with enticing decisions.

7. Time Usage Difficulties:

Issue:

Battling to carve out opportunities for feast planning and exercise.

Arrangement:

Focus on your timetable, plan dinners ahead of time, and investigate fast, nutritious recipes. Integrate short eruptions of actual work over the day, guaranteeing you stay dynamic notwithstanding a bustling timetable.

8. Undesirable Desires:

Issue:

Managing steady desires for unfortunate food sources.

Arrangement:

Distinguish triggers for desires and supplant unfortunate choices with nutritious other options. Guarantee your feasts are even, and consider counseling a nutritionist for customized techniques.

9. Overtraining:

Issue:

Encountering weakness, absence of progress, or expanded hazard of injury because of over-the-top activity.

Arrangement:

Permit satisfactory rest days, differ your gym routine daily schedule, and focus on recuperation rehearses like extending or yoga. Higher standards no matter what are key in accomplishing supportable wellness.

10. Unreasonable Assumptions:

Issue:

Putting forth excessively aggressive or impossible objectives.

Arrangement:

Lay out reasonable, quantifiable objectives and celebrate accomplishments en route. Comprehend that the Full Body Reset is an excursion, and feasible advancement takes time.

Adjusting the Full Body Reset program for lactose-bigoted older people requires smart thought to guarantee ideal well-being and adherence. Here is a custom-made way to deal with obliging their necessities:

1. Without dairy Protein Sources: Older people with lactose bigotry can in any case meet their protein needs through elective sources. Consolidate lean meats, poultry, fish, eggs, and plant-based protein choices like tofu, tempeh, and vegetables. These options give fundamental amino acids to muscle maintenance and general well-being.

2. Plant-Based Milk Options: Supplant customary dairy with sans lactose or plant-based milk options like almond, coconut, or oat milk. These choices are generally accessible and give a supplement-rich base to smoothies, cereals, and different recipes. Guarantee the chosen options are braced with fundamental supplements like calcium and vitamin D.

3. Sans lactose Dairy Items: Investigate without lactose forms of dairy items like yogurt and cheddar. Numerous general stores offer sans-lactose options that hold the taste and wholesome advantages of customary dairy without causing stomach-related uneasiness.

4. Center around Absorbable Entire Food varieties: Underline entire, effectively edible food sources in the feast plan. Integrate cooked vegetables, very much cooked grains, and effectively absorbable proteins to diminish the weight on the stomach-related framework.

5. Probiotic-rich food varieties: While customary yogurt might be off the table, lactose-bigoted people can in any case profit from probiotics. Incorporate matured food varieties like sauerkraut, kimchi, and sans lactose yogurt choices to help stomach wellbeing.

6. Screen Fiber Admission: Focus on fiber admission, as some high-fiber food sources can add to gas and swelling. Steadily present fiber-rich food sources, like organic products, vegetables, and entire grains, to permit the stomach-related framework to adjust.

7. Satisfactory Hydration: Guarantee adequate hydration, particularly while consolidating fiber-rich food sources. Water and homegrown teas can help absorption and forestall drying out, especially significant for the old populace.

8. Customized Dinner Arranging: Tailor the Full Body Reset dinner plans to individual inclinations and resilience. Consider talking with an enrolled dietitian or nutritionist to make a customized dinner plan that lines up with the program's standards while obliging lactose prejudice.

9. Delicate Activity Choices: Recognize potential portability challenges in old people and proposition delicate activity choices. Exercises like strolling, swimming, or seat activities can add to generally speaking prosperity without putting excessive weight on joints.

10. Standard Observing and Variation: Routinely screen the singular's reaction to dietary changes and exercise. Adjust the program depending on the situation given criticism, making acclimations to upgrade solace and adherence.

Defeating profound eating and pigging out among the older requires a smart and steady methodology. Here are a few procedures to assist with tending to these difficulties:

1. Recognize Triggers:

- Urge self-reflection to distinguish triggers for profound or gorging. This mindfulness is vital for creating powerful survival methods.

2. Basic encouragement:

- Cultivate a strong climate, empowering open correspondence. Forlornness or stress can be critical triggers, so having areas of strength for a framework is indispensable.

3. Take part in Friendly Exercises:

- Empower cooperation in friendly exercises to battle segregation. This can incorporate local area occasions, clubs, or investing energy with loved ones.

4. Energize Close to home Articulation:

- Advance solid approaches to communicating feelings, for example, journaling, workmanship, or participating in exercises that give pleasure and satisfaction.

5. Careful Eating Practices:

- Support careful eating by focusing on appetite and completion signs. Urge the old to enjoy each chomp and eat without interruptions.

6. Adjusted Nourishment:

- Guarantee that the older are getting an even eating routine to address dietary issues. Lacks of specific supplements can add to close to home eating.

7. Customary Dinner Times:

- Lay out customary dinner times to give design and solidness. This can assist with forestalling imprudent eating beyond arranged feasts.

8. Look for Proficient Assistance:

- Energize looking for help from medical care experts, including advisors, dietitians, or therapists who work in profound eating.

9. Make a Place of refuge:

- Establish a climate where it is invited to talk about profound worries. Having a good sense of reassurance to communicate feelings can assist with lessening the requirement for profound eating as a survival technique.

10. Foster Survival methods:

- Help with creating elective survival techniques for stress or close to home trouble, like profound breathing activities, reflection, or taking part in leisure activities.

11. Gradual Methodology:

- Support continuous changes. Handy solutions may not be economical, and a gradual methodology frequently yields additional enduring outcomes.

12. Empower Actual work:

- Advance delicate actual work customized to individual capacities. The practice has a state of mind helping impacts and can act as a constructive option for stress.

13. Screen Prescriptions:

- Work intimately with medical services experts to screen meds that might impact craving or mindset. Changes might be important.

14. Help to remember Past Triumphs:

- Help the old to remember past victories and survival techniques they've utilized successfully. This builds up their capacity to beat difficulties.

15. Energize a Positive Relationship with Food:

- Cultivate a positive relationship with food by underlining its part in sustenance and pleasure as opposed to involving it as a wellspring of solace.

Adjusting the Full Body Reset for older people confronting difficulties with consuming leafy foods requires a careful and steady methodology. Here are methodologies to address troubles in consolidating these fundamental parts:

1. Smoothies and Mixed Soups:

Make supplement-loaded smoothies by mixing natural products with non-dairy options, for example, almond or coconut milk. Additionally, get ready to mix soups with vegetables to make them simpler to consume. This approach holds the nourishing substance while tending to surface worries.

2. Cooked or Steamed Choices:

Pick cooked or steamed vegetables rather than crude, as they are many times milder and gentler on the stomach-related framework. Explore different avenues regarding different cooking strategies to upgrade flavor and make them engaging.

3. Try different things with Flavors:

Improve the flavor of products of the soil by exploring different avenues regarding spices, flavors, and flavors. This can make them more satisfactory and agreeable, empowering normal utilization.

4. Assortment of Planning Techniques:

Offer various planning techniques for products of the soil to take care of various inclinations. Simmering, barbecuing, sautéing, or pan-searing can bring out one-of-a-kind flavors and surfaces that may more allure.

5. Remember for Most loved Dishes:

Incorporate products of the soil into recognizable dishes that the individual appreciates. For instance, add finely slashed vegetables to meals, omelets, or pasta dishes, or integrate natural products into yogurt or entire grain oat.

6. Soups and Stews:

Get ready to supplement rich soups and stews with a blend of vegetables and lean proteins. The cooking system relaxes the vegetables, making them simpler to bite and process while giving fundamental supplements.

7. Pre-sliced and Prepared to-Eat Choices:

Make products of the soil more open by pre-cutting them into reduced down pieces. Having prepared-to-eat choices promptly accessible can take out hindrances and support customary utilization.

8. Continuous Presentation:

Present products of the soil progressively, beginning with little parcels. Permit time for the taste buds to adjust, and energize attempting new choices occasionally to grow the range of food sources eaten.

9. Supplement Thick Tidbits:

Integrate supplement thick bites that join natural products or vegetables with protein or solid fats. Models incorporate apple cuts with almond spread or carrot sticks with hummus.

10. Counsel with a Nutritionist:

Consider talking with a nutritionist or dietitian who has some expertise in old sustenance. They can give customized direction, address explicit worries, and make a custom-made plan that lines up with the Full Body Reset standards.

11. Hydration with Injected Water:

Support hydration by imbuing water with cuts of natural products or spices. This adds an unpretentious flavor and can be a charming method for expanding liquid admission, particularly if plain water is less engaging.

Adjusting the Full Body Reset for old people, particularly those confronting difficulties in consuming products of the soil, requires a patient and adaptable methodology. By carrying out custom-made methodologies, a modified program can be made to help ideal well-being while at the same time thinking about individual inclinations and impediments. Perceiving the uniqueness of every individual and looking for proficient direction cultivates a merciful and strong climate, imperative for defeating difficulties in the excursion toward a trim figure and ideal well-being. Similar standards apply while tending to lactose narrow-mindedness, guaranteeing a strong and comprehensive methodology for a positive and economical involvement with the Full Body Reset program.

Summary

"The Full Body Reset" is an extensive aide intended to engage people on their extraordinary excursion to weight reduction, ideal well-being, and a body they'll cherish into midlife. The book unpredictably explores key standards like careful nourishment, designated exercise, and way of life changes. From understanding the complexities of stomach well-being to investigating normal difficulties, the book gives functional answers for maintainable advancement. Customized guidance for explicit populaces, like the old or those with lactose prejudice, guarantees inclusivity. With an emphasis on steady changes, customized techniques, and a comprehensive methodology, "The Full Body Reset" fills in as a guide to accomplish a trim figure as well as to develop long-lasting propensities that encourage prosperity and essentialness.